Definitive guide to Sirtfood Diet

Healthy Recipes to Activate Your Skinny Gene and Burn Fat, Lose Weight, and Eat Healthier with Exclusive Recipes Preparations for Your Meal Plan

Lisa T. Oliver

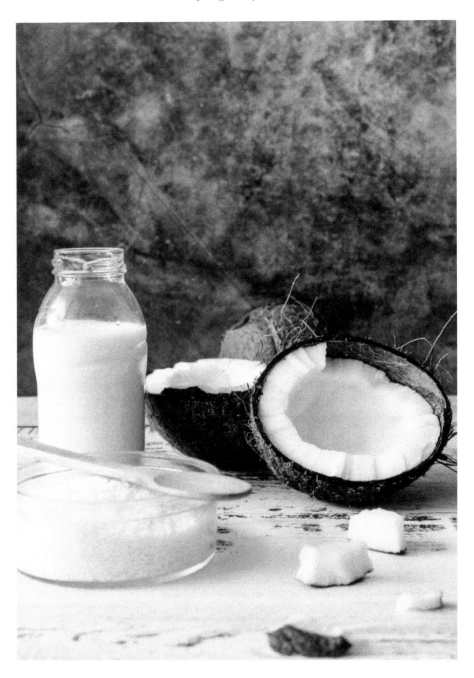

Table Of Contents

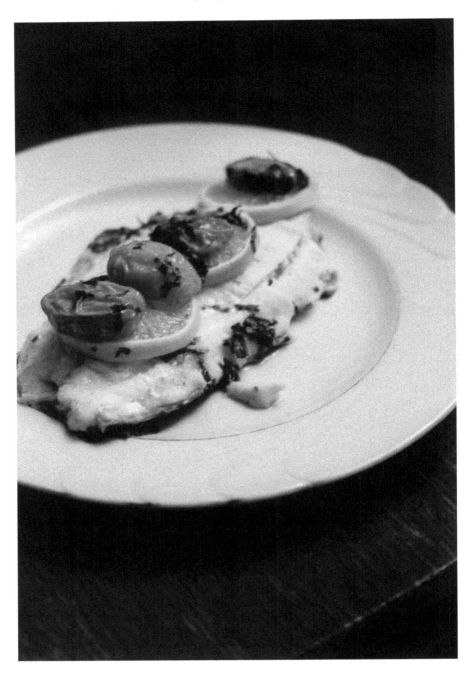

Introduction

The Sirtfood Diet, launched in 2016, has been a trending topic for a while now, with people following the diet very strictly. The creators of the diet suggest that these foods function by activating proteins in the body, referred to as sirtuins. The idea is that sirtuins protect body cells from dying when subjected to stress and regulate metabolism, inflammation, and aging. Sirtuins also boost the body's metabolism and affect its ability to burn fat, providing a weight loss of about seven pounds in a week while retaining muscle. Nonetheless, experts believe that this is solely about fat loss rather than differences in glycogen storage from the liver and skeletal muscle. This diet was developed by UK-based nutritionists, both with MAs in nutritional medicine, and has since gained popularity among athletes and celebrities. Adele and Pippa Middleton are two celebrities who have followed the Sirtfood Diet, and it yielded great results for them. The Sirtfood Diet, like most diets, promotes sustained and significant weight loss, improved health, and better energy. What is it about this diet? Is it just a fad, or is there more to it? Does science back it up? All these questions and more will be answered as you read on. The word "sirt" comes from sirtuins, a group of Silent Information Regulator (SIR) proteins. They boost metabolism, improve muscle efficiency, reduce inflammation, and start the process of fat loss and cell repair. These sirtuins make us healthier, fit, and also help in fighting diseases. Exercise and restrictions on calorie consumption improve sirtuin production in the body.

What Are Sirtfoods?

About the Sirtfood Diet

The Sirtfood Diet plan considers that some foods activate your "skinny gene" and can make you lose about seven pounds in about a week.Certain foods, such as dark chocolate, kale, and wine, contain polyphenols, a natural chemical that imitates exercise and fasting and affects the body. Other sirtfoods include cinnamon, red onions, and turmeric. These trigger the sirtuins' pathway and start weight loss. There is scientific evidence to support this too. The impact of weight loss is higher in the first week. The Sirtfood Diet mainly consists of plant-based foods that are rich in sirtuins to trigger fat loss. The diet is divided into two phases, which can be repeated continuously. The first phase is three days of living on 1000 calories and four days of 1500 calories with lots of green juices.

The Premise of the Sirtfood Diet The premise of the Sirtfood Diet states that certain foods can mimic the benefits of fasting and caloric restrictions by activating sirtuins, which are proteins in the body. They range from SIRT1 to SIRT7, switch genes on and off, maintain biological pathways, and protect cells from age-related decline. Although intense calorie restriction and fasting are severe, the Sirtfood Diet inventors developed a plan with a focus on eating plenty of sirtfoods. It's a more natural way to stimulate sirtuin genes in the body, also known as skinny genes. In the process, it improves health and boosts weight loss. If you want to start the Sirtfood Diet, planning is required, and access to the ingredients needed to follow the diet correctly. There are many exciting recipes for the diet, with a variety of ingredients. However, it may often be challenging to get certain ingredients during specific seasons and times of the year. Some of these ingredients include kale and strawberries, for example. It may also be stressful to follow social events when traveling or to care for a young child. The Sirtfood Diet covers various food groups; however, dairy foods aren't included in the plan. Sirtfoods are a new diet discovery. They are rich in nutrients and capable of activating skinny genes in the body, with benefits and downsides alike.

CHAPTER 1:

Breakfast

1.   Cobb Salad

Preparation Time: 10 minutes

Cooking Time: 30 minutes

Servings: 4

Ingredients

Four slices of bacon

Four eggs

1/4 cup blue (icing)

1/2 cup cherry tomatoes (leave whole)

2 cups cucumbers (chopped)

4 cups romaine lettuce (Washed, cracked, and dried)

Red Wine Vinaigrette

Two tablespoons wine vinegar

Two tablespoons extra virgin vegetable oil

1 tbsp. honey (or maple syrup; see low carb *)

1/4 teaspoon Dijon mustard

salt and pepper

optional - fresh

Add one avocado (chopped)

green onion (chopped)

Directions:

While cooking the bacon inside a frying pan or oven, keep aside cool and dig small pieces.

Cook eggs in a pot or on the stove. Let it cool. Peel and dig cubes.

Prep the wine vinaigrette and toss all the vegetables within the dressing.

Divide vegetables between four bowls. Hard-coded egg, blue, avocado, and chives if desired, with bacon.

A multi-compartm nt container keeps the veggies away from the dressing (I further.

Keep in an airtight container in the fridge for four days.

Enjoy all the ingredients before serving!

Use a spice container for stuffing). I like to keep my eggs peeled, but you will peel them

2.   Western Wild Rice And Sweet Salad

Preparation Time: 10 minutes

Cooking Time: 30 minutes

Servings: 4

Ingredients

Roasted Sweet Potatoes

4 cups sweet potatoes (peeled and dug 1-inch cubes, roughly one big or two small sweet potatoes)

One teaspoon vegetable oil

incense shade

salad

3/4 cup wild rice mixture (Uncooked)

One carrot (peeled and grated)

One celery (finely chopped)

One red chili (diced)

One yellow pepper (diced)

1/4 cup purple onion (finely chopped)

1/2 cup cilantro leaves (approx. fully sliced; loosely packed).

Vinaigrette

3tablespoons vegetable oil

Three tablespoons wine vinegar

Two teaspoons juice

One teaspoon taste

Two teaspoons honey (maple syrup makes it vegetarian)

One clove garlic (minced)

1/4 teaspoon salt

Directions:

Roasted sweet potato

Heat oven 425 ° F. Season with sweet protein vegetable oil and salt and pepper. Arrange on a baking sheet or baking dish.

Bake for quarter-hours, stirring, and still bake for 10–15 minutes until the fork easily comes from the sweet potato. Remove from the oven and set aside fresh.

The Salad

The Cook Rice package conforms to the instructions. You should only find yourself with 2 cups of cooked rice. Let the salad cool completely before assembling.

Combine cooled sweet potato, cooked rice, and remaining salad ingredients.

Stir all the vinaigrette ingredients together and toss the salad well.

Storage

If you are getting the salad, make-ahead, leave the cilantro until just before serving.

Flap for food - discard the cilantro and add a can of black beans. Sh2 cups in a food prep container and refrigerate for four days.

3.   Kale Caesar Salad

Preparation Time: 10 minutes

Cooking Time: 20 minutes

Servings: 4

Ingredients

Garlic Peel Garlic Peel

19 oz. Cooked chickpeas (dry and rotten; about 2 cups)

One tablespoon arrowroot starch (or all-purpose flour)

Two tablespoons garlic powder

1/2 teaspoon salt tsp.

3Spoon Vegetable Oil

Greek Yogurt Caesar Dressing:

1/4 cup Greek Yogurt

1/4 cup Avocado Mayonnaise (or your favorite mayo)

One teaspoon Flavoring

Four teaspoons Rasch Mac

2 Cloves Garlic (minced)

Pepper

Chickpea Black Salad: Banana

1 (washed, Chopped, and dried)

1/4 cup Parmesan. Paneer (sliced)

Directions:

Roast the garlic peel and then spread them on a clean towel and blot with a second towel dry thoroughly. Once the chickpeas dry shake them until evenly coated with arrowroot starch, garlic powder, and salt. Heat oil in a pan on medium heat. Add the chickpeas to the pan and cook for 15-20 minutes until they golden brown. Remove slightly from heat and funky. Keel Caesar salad kale

While garlic chickpeas for cooking, slicing, washing, and drying.

Stir the dressing ingredients together, and then toss until the bud is evenly coated.

Serve

Keel Caesar Salad with Garlic Chole and a tablespoon of Parmesan Cheese

eat the recipe

The salad best served fresh, although you have several ingredients ready after 4-5 days

will- Shred, wash in a while in a container lined with dry towel within the fridge -

Stir store fridge kale handshake and store.

4.   Pineapple Buckle Pancake

Preparation Time: 10 minutes

Cooking Time: 30 minutes

Servings: 4

Ingredients

1 cup cereal flour

1/4 cup almond flour

2 tbsp. asafetida seeds, plus toppings For

One teaspoon. Yeast

1/2 teaspoon allspice

1/4 teaspoon salt

Pineapple Mauna Pot Cheese 5.3 oz.

One egg

Two tablespoons syrup, services for more

One teaspoon vanilla

1 cup sweet almond milk (or other milk)

plus, one small pineapple, outer Flake in chopped rings and cored, (you can also use canned pineapple rings)

1tbsp butter, split

Directions:

Heat a pancake grill or pan over medium heat.

Combine flour, hemp seeds, yeast, allspice, and salt during a large bowl and whisk until combined.

Add pot cheese, egg, syrup, vanilla to the bowl. Slowly add everything until you add the milk gradually.

Add a little butter to the pan. Once melted, place a pineapple ring on top and cook until golden brown and begin caramelizing. Flip the pineapple slices over, pour the spoon batter over it to cover the ring completely, and touch the edges. Cook until set (about 3 minutes), flip carefully, and cook for 2 minutes on the other side.

Repeat with remaining pineapple rings and batter.

Serve with syrup and extra hemp seeds for topping.

5.   Crude Brownie Bites

Preparation Time: 10 minutes

Cooking Time: 5 minutes

Servings: 6

Ingredients:

2½ cups entire walnuts

¼ cup almonds

2½ cups Medjool dates

1 cup cacao powder

1 teaspoon vanilla concentrate

⅛-¼ teaspoon ocean salt

Directions:

Spot everything in a nourishment processor until very much joined.

Fold into balls and spot on a heating sheet and freeze for 30 minutes or refrigerate for 2 hours.

  Nutrition:

Energy (calories): 1677 kcal

Protein: 47.18 g

Fat: 141.93 g Carbohydrates: 123.14 g

6.　　Potato Salad

Time: 15 minutes

Cooking Time: 0 minutes

Servings: 2

Ingredients:

200g celery, generally slashed

100g apple, typically slashed

50g walnuts, generally slashed

1 little red onion, generally slashed

1 head of chicory, slashed

10g level parsley, slashed

1 tbsp. escapades

10g lovage or celery leaves, typically slashed

For the dressing:

1 tbsp. additional virgin olive oil

1 tsp. balsamic vinegar

1 teaspoon Dijon mustard

Juice of a large portion of a lemon

Directions:

Blend the celery, apple, walnuts, onion, parsley, escapades, and lavage/celery in a medium-sized plate of mixed greens bowl and blend.

Make the dressing by whisking together the oil, vinegar, mustard, and lemon juice. Drizzle over the plate of mixed greens, blend and serve!

Nutrition:

Energy (calories): 542 kcal

Protein: 11.74 g

Fat: 39.66 g

Carbohydrates: 44.44 g

7. Chargrilled Beef With A Red Wine Jus, Onion Rings, Garlic, Kale And Herb Roasted Potatoes

Preparation Time: 10 minutes

Cooking Time: 40 minutes

Servings: 4

Ingredients:

100g potatoes, stripped and cut into 2cm bones

1 tbsp. additional virgin olive oil

5g parsley, finely hacked

50g red onion, cut into rings

50g kale, cut

1 garlic clove, finely hacked

120–150g x 3.5cm-thick meat filet steak or 2cm-thick sirloin steak

40ml red wine

150ml meat stock

1 tsp. tomato purée

1 tsp. Corn flour broke up in 1 tbsp. water

Directions:

Heat the oven to 220°C/gas 7.

Spot the potatoes in a pot of boiling water, take back to the boil and cook for 4–5 minutes at that point channel. A spot in a simmering tin with one teaspoon of the oil and dish in the hot stove for 35–45 minutes. Turn the potatoes like clockwork to guarantee, in any event, cooking. When cooked, expel from the oven, sprinkle with the hacked parsley and blend well.

Fry the onion in 1 teaspoon of the oil over medium heat for 5–7 minutes, until delicate and pleasantly caramelized. Keep warm. Steam the kale for 2–3 minutes at that point channel. Fry the garlic tenderly in ½ teaspoon of oil for one moment, until delicate yet not shaded. Include the kale and fry for a further 1–2 minutes, until tender. Keep warm.

Heat an ovenproof skillet over high heat until smoking. Coat the meat in ½ a teaspoon of the oil and fry in the hot skillet over medium-high heat as indicated by how you like your heart done. If you want your meat medium, it is smarter to burn the meat and afterward move the container to a stove set at 220°C/gas 7 and finish the cooking that path for the endorsed occasions. Expel the meat from the dish and put it aside to rest. Add the wine to the hot skillet to raise any meat buildup— air pocket to considerably lessen the wine until syrupy and with a concentrated flavor. Include the stock and tomato purée to the steak container and bring to the boil; at that point, add the cornflour glue to thicken your sauce, including it a little at once until you have your ideal consistency. Mix in any of the juices from the refreshed steak and present with the broiled potatoes, kale, onion rings, and red wine sauce.

8.   New Saag Paneer

Preparation Time: 10 minutes

Cooking Time: 30 minutes

Servings: 2

Ingredients:

2 tsp. rapeseed oil

200g paneer.

Cut into 3D shapes

Salt and crisply ground dark pepper

One red onion, cleaved

One little thumb (3 cm) new ginger, stripped and cut into matchsticks

One clove garlic, stripped and daintily cut

One green bean stew, deseeded and finely cut

100g cherry tomatoes, split

1/2 tsp. ground coriander

1/2 tsp. ground cumin

1/4 tsp. ground turmeric

1/2 tsp. gentle stew powder

1/2 tsp. salt

100g new spinach leaves

Little bunch (10g) parsley, cleaved

Small bunch (10g) coriander, cleaved

Directions:

Heat the oil in a vast, lidded skillet over high heat. Season the paneer liberally with salt and pepper and hurl it into the dish. Fry for a couple of moments until brilliant, blending regularly. Expel from the plate with an opened spoon and put in a safe spot.

Reduce the heat and include the onion. Fry for 5 minutes before having the ginger, garlic, and stew. Cook for another couple of minutes before having the cherry tomatoes. Put the top on the dish and cook for a further 5 minutes.

Add the flavors and salt; at that point, mix. Return the paneer to the dish and mix until covered. Add the spinach to the container together with the parsley and coriander and put the cover on. Permit the spinach to fade for 1-2 minutes. At that point, consolidate into the dish. Serve right away.

Nutrition:

Energy (calories): 422 kcal

Protein: 15.6 g Fat: 23.57 g

Carbohydrates: 43.7 g

9. Mocha Chocolate Mousse

Preparation Time: 10 minutes

Cooking Time: 130 minutes

Servings: 4-6

Everybody appreciates chocolate mousse, and this one has a brilliant light and breezy surface. It is brisk and straightforward to make and is best served the day after it's made.

Ingredients:

- 250g dim chocolate (85% cocoa solids)

- 6 medium unfenced eggs, isolated

- 4 tbsp. solid dark espresso

- 4 tbsp. almond milk

- Chocolate espresso beans, to enrich

Directions:

Soften the chocolate in a vast bowl set over a skillet of delicately stewing water, ensuring the bowl's base doesn't contact the water. Expel the bowl from the heat and leave the dissolved chocolate to cool to room temperature.

When the softened chocolate is at room temperature, race in the egg yolks each in turn and afterward tenderly overlap in the espresso and almond milk.

Utilizing a hand-held electric blender, whisk the egg whites until firm pinnacles structure; at that point, blend several tablespoons into the chocolate blend to release it. Delicately overlap in the rest of a giant metal spoon. Move the mousse to special glasses and smooth the surface. Spread with stick film and chill for in any event 2 hours, preferably medium-term. Enliven with chocolate espresso beans before serving.

Nutrition:

Energy (calories): 1110 kcal

Protein: 38.86 g Fat: 28.79 g

Carbohydrates: 171.28 g

10.   Buckwheat Superfood Muesli

Preparation Time: 10 minutes

Cooking Time: 0 minutes

Servings: 4

Ingredients:

- 20g buckwheat pieces

- 10g buckwheat puffs

- 15g coconut pieces or parched coconut

- 40g Medjool dates, hollowed and cleaved

- 15g walnuts, cleaved

- 10g cocoa nibs

- 100g strawberries, hulled and cleaved

- 100g plain Greek yogurt (or veggie lover elective, for example, soy or coconut yogurt)

Directions:

Blend the entirety of the above Ingredients: together (forget about the strawberries and yogurt if not serving straight away).

If you need to make this in mass or set it up the previous night, just join the dry Ingredients: and store it in an impenetrable holder. All you have to do the following day is include the strawberries and yogurt, and it is all set.

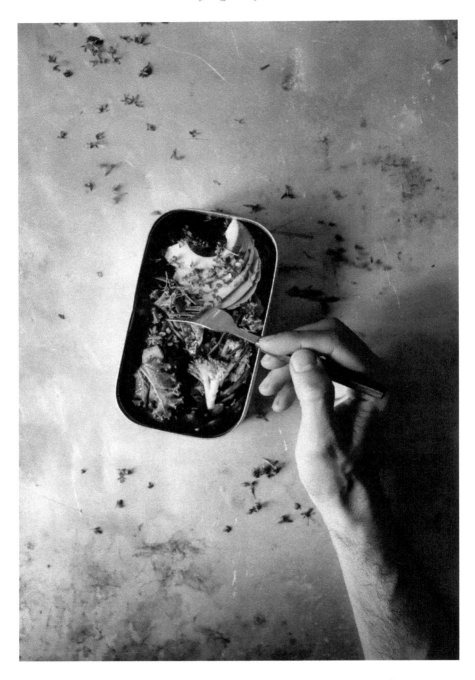

CHAPTER 2:

Lunch

11.   Chicken Curry Pasta

Preparation time: 10 minutes

Cooking time: 2hours to4 hours

Servings: 4

Ingredients:

500 g chicken breast

Teaspoon of paprika

Onion slices

Clove garlic

One teaspoon of clarified butter

Spoon curry powder

500ml coconut milk (box)

200g pineapple

200g mango

chili

Pumpkin

25 g shallots

25 grams of fresh coriander

Directions:

Cut the chicken into strips and season with pepper, salt, and pepper. Then put the chicken in the slow cooker.

Finely chop the onion and garlic, then gently sauté with two teaspoons of clarified butter. Then add curry powder.

Add coconut milk frosting after one minute. Put soy sauce in a slow cooker with pineapple, mango slices, chopped peppers, and cook for 2 to 4 hours.

Slice the pumpkin into thin slices and use a screwdriver to slice the pasta into thin slices (not easy, it is best to use carrots).

Fry the pumpkin spaghetti briefly in the pan, then sprinkle the chicken curry on top.

Garnish with chopped green onions and chopped cilantro.

Nutrition:

Energy (calories): 1172 kcal

Protein: 108.54 g

Fat: 51.46 g Carbohydrates: 69.55 g

12.   French Chicken Thighs

Preparation time: 10 minutes

Cooking time: 4 hours and 15 minutes Servings: 4

Ingredients:

700g chicken thighs

A spoon of olive oil

Onion slices

radish

Garlic clove

8 Celery

25g fresh rosemary

25g fresh thyme

Directions:

Prepare 25 grams of fresh parsleySeason the chicken with olive oil, pepper, and salt, and then knead it into the meat.Finely chop onions, carrots, garlic, and celery and place in a slow cooker. Place the chicken on top and sprinkle a few drops of rosemary, thyme, and parsley on top—Cook for at least four hours.Serve with a delicious salad and enjoy the food! Nutrition:Energy (calories): 1674 kcal Protein: 120.18 g Fat: 118.52 g Carbohydrates: 28.73 g

13.   Thai Vegetarian Green Curry

Preparation time: 15 minutes

Cooking time: 4hours and 20 minutes

Servings: 4

Ingredients:

green pepper

Onion slices

Clove garlic

Teaspoon fresh ginger (ground)

25 grams fresh coriander

One teaspoon coriander

One portion of lemon juice

One teaspoon coconut oil

500 ml of coconut milk

One zucchini slice

One-piece broccoli

One red pepper

For cauliflower rice:

One teaspoon coconut oil

One cauliflower

Directions:

For the cauliflower rice, cut the cauliflower into florets and put them in a food processor. Stir briefly until rice forms. Put on hold. Cut green peppers, onions, garlic, fresh ginger, and coriander into small pieces, mix them with coriander seeds, and lime juice in a food processor or blender. Heat a teaspoon of coconut oil on medium heat and fry the paste lightly. Freeze coconut milk and heat over low heat.

Cut the zucchini into thin slices, cut the broccoli into florets, cut the peppers into small pieces, and then put them in a slow cooker—Cook for 4 hours.

Heat cauliflower rice briefly in 1 teaspoon of coconut oil, add a little salt and pepper to the pot.

Nutrition:

Energy (calories): 141 kcal

Protein: 2.89 g

Fat: 9.61 g

Carbohydrates: 14.96 g

14.   Indian Yellow Curry

Preparation time: 10 minutes

Cooking time: 20minutes

Servings: 4

Ingredients:

Onion slices

One clove garlic

300 g chicken breast

A teaspoon of coconut oil

One tablespoon curry powder

One teaspoon fresh ginger

One teaspoon turmeric

One teaspoon

500ml coconut milk salad:

250 g iceberg lettuce

/ 2 slices of cucumber

A piece of bell pepper

25 grams dry parsley

Directions:

Heat the pot on medium heat to dissolve the coconut oil.

Finely chop onion and garlic. Put in the pot; add herbs, icing sugar, and coconut milk, mix well.

Cut the chicken into small pieces and put them in a slow cooker together with curry.

Shred the iceberg lettuce, sprinkle with cucumber and pepper slices, and season with coriander. Drink salad and curry together.

Nutrition:

Energy (calories): 719 kcal

Protein: 75.21 g

Fat: 35.06

Carbohydrates: 31.4 g

15.   Sticky Chicken Water Melon Noodle Salad

Preparation time: 10 minutes

Cooking time: 25 minutes

Servings: 4

Ingredients

Two pieces of skinny rice noodles

1/2 Tbsp. sesame oil

2 cups Water Melon

Head of bib lettuce

Half of a Lot of scallions

Half of a Lot of fresh cilantro

Two skinless, boneless chicken breasts

1/2 Tbsp. Chinese five-spice

1 Tbsp. Extra virgin olive oil

two Tbsp. sweet skillet (I utilized a mixture of maple syrup using a dash of Tabasco)

1 Tbsp. sesame seeds

a couple of cashews - smashed

Dressing - could be made daily or two until

1 Tbsp. low-salt soy sauce

One teaspoon sesame oil

1 Tbsp. peanut butter

Half of a refreshing red chili

Half of a couple of chives

Half of a couple of cilantro

One lime - juiced

One small spoonful of garlic

Directions:

At a bowl, then completely substituting the noodles in boiling drinking water. They are going to be soon carried out in 2 minutes.

On a big parchment paper sheet, throw the chicken with pepper, salt, and the five-spice.

Twist over the newspaper, subsequently celebrate, and put the chicken using a rolling pin.

Place into the large skillet with 1 Tbsp. Of olive oil, she is turning 3 or 4 minutes, until well charred and cooked through.

Drain the noodles and toss with 1 Tbsp. Of sesame oil onto a sizable serving dish.

Place 50% of the noodles into the medium skillet, frequently stirring until crispy and nice.

Eliminate the Watermelon skin, then slice the flesh to inconsistent balls and then increase the platter.

Reduce the lettuces and cut into small wedges and half of many leafy greens and scatter the dish.

Place another 1 / 2 the cilantro pack, soy sauce, coriander, chives, peanut butter, a dab of water, one teaspoon of sesame oil, and the lime juice mix till smooth.

Set the chicken back to heat, garnish with the entire sweet skillet (or my walnut syrup mixture), and toss with the sesame seeds.

Pour the dressing on the salad, toss gently with fresh fingers until well coated, add crispy noodles, and smash cashews.

Blend chicken pieces and add them to the salad.

16.   Fruity Curry Chicken Salad

Preparation time: 10 minutes Cooking time: 15 minutes

Servings: 4 Ingredients

Four skinless, boneless Chicken Pliers - cooked and diced

1 tsp. celery, diced

Four green onions, sliced

1 Golden Delicious apple peeled, cored, and diced

1/3 cup golden raisins

1/3 cup seedless green grapes, halved

1/2 cup sliced toasted pecans

$\frac{1}{8}$ teaspoon ground black pepper

1/2 tsp. curry powder

3/4 cup light mayonnaise

Directions:

Measure 1

In a big bowl, combine the chicken, onion, celery, apple, celery, celery, pecans, pepper, curry powder, and carrot. Mix altogether. Drink!

Nutrition: Energy (calories): 1223 kcal Protein: 18.21 g Fat: 93.59 g Carbohydrates: 88.9 g

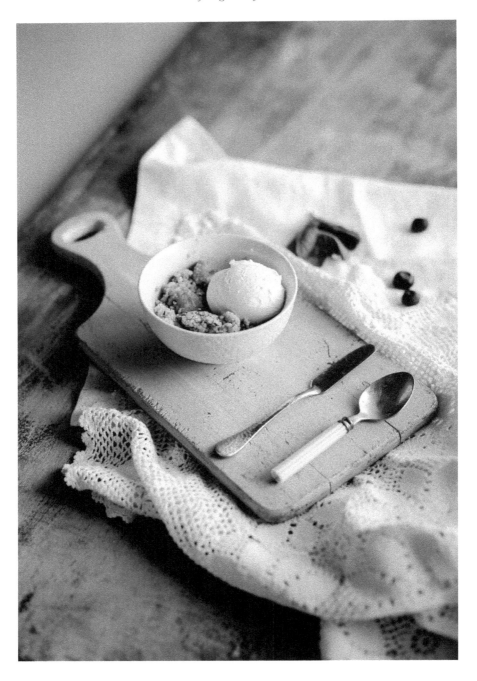

CHAPTER 3:

Dinner

17.   Protein Power Sweet Potatoes

Preparation Time: 1hr

Cooking Time: 40 to 45 minutes

Servings: 2 servings

Ingredients:

Two medium sweet potatoes 6 ounces plain Greek yogurt

½ teaspoon salt 1/3 cup dried cranberries

¼ teaspoon freshly ground black pepper

Directions:

Heat. The oven to 400 degrees F and pierce the sweet potatoes several times. Place them on a cooking plate and cook for 40 to 45 minutes, or until you can easily pierce them with a fork. Cut the potatoes in half and wrap the meat in a medium bowl and keep the skin healthy. Add the salt, pepper, yogurt, and cranberries to the pan and mix well with a fork. Spoon the mixture back into the potato skins and serve warm.

Nutrition: Fat 11g, Carbohydrates 15g, and Protein 18g

18.   Penne Pasta With Vegetables

Preparation Time: 15 minutes

Cooking Time: 9 minutes

Servings: 2 servings

Ingredients:

One teaspoon salt, divided ¾ cup uncooked penne pasta

One tablespoon olive oil One tablespoon chopped garlic

One teaspoon chopped fresh oregano 1 cup sliced fresh mushrooms to cherry tomatoes, halved

1 cup fresh spinach leaves ½ teaspoon freshly ground black pepper

One tablespoon shredded Parmesan cheese

Directions:

In a large saucepan, bring 1-quart water to a boil. Add 1/2 teaspoon of the salt and the penne, and cook according to package directions or until al dente (about 9 minutes). Drain but do not rinse the penne, reserving about VA cup pasta water. Meanwhile, in a large skillet, heat the olive oil over medium-high heat. Add the garlic, oregano, mushrooms, and sauté for 4 to 5 minutes, or until the mushrooms are golden.

Add the tomatoes and spinach, season with the remaining ½ teaspoon salt and the black pepper, and sauté for 3 to 4 minutes, or until the spinach is wilted.

Add the drained pasta to the skillet, along with 2 to 3 tablespoons of the pasta water. Cook, constantly stirring, for 2 to 3 minutes, or until the pasta is glistening and the water has cooked off. Divide the pasta between two shallow bowls and sprinkle with the Parmesan cheese. Serve hot or at room temperature.

Nutrition: Fat 12g, Carbohydrates 9g, and Protein 19g

19.   Spinach And Swiss Cheese Omelet

Preparation Time: 5 minutes

Cooking Time: 3 to 4 minutes

Servings: 2 servings

Ingredients:

One teaspoon olive oil Six large egg whites, beaten

1 cup fresh baby spinach leaves 2 (1-ounce) slices reduced-fat Swiss cheese

½ teaspoon salt

¼ teaspoon freshly ground black pepper

Directions:

In a small skillet, heat the olive oil over medium-high heat. Add the spinach, salt, and pepper, and sauté for 3 minutes, stirring often.

Use a spatula to spread the spinach reasonably evenly over the pan's bottom and pour the egg whites over the top, tilting the pan to coat the spinach thoroughly.

Cook for 3 to 4 minutes, occasionally pulling the edges of the eggs toward the center as you thrust the skillet to allow uncooked egg to spread to the sides of the pan. When the eggs' centers are mostly (but not wholly) dry, use a spatula to flip the eggs. Place the Swiss cheese slices on one half of the omelet, and then scan the other half over the top to form a half-moon. Cook for 1 minute, or until the cheese is melted and warm. To serve, cut the omelet in half and serve hot.

Nutrition:

Fat 8g, Carbohydrates 12g, and Protein 18g

20. Broiled Halibut With Garlic Spinach

Preparation Time: 7 to 8 minutes

Cooking Time: 6 to 7 minutes

Servings: 2 servings

Ingredients:

2 (4-ounce) halibut fillets, 1-inch thick ½ lemon (about one teaspoon juice)

One teaspoon salt, divided ¼ teaspoon freshly ground black pepper

½ teaspoon cayenne pepper 1 teaspoon olive oil Two cloves garlic

½ cup chopped red onion

2 cups fresh baby spinach leaves

Directions:

Preheat the broiler and place an oven rack 4 to 5 inches below the heat source. Line a baking sheet with aluminum foil.

Squeeze the lemon half over the fish fillets, and then season each side with ½ teaspoon of salt, pepper, and cayenne. Place the fish on the pan and broil for 7 to 8 minutes. Turn over the fish and cook for 6 to 7 minutes more, or until flaky.

Meanwhile, heat the olive oil in a small skillet over medium heat. Add the garlic and onion, and sauté for 2 minutes. Add the spinach and remaining ½ teaspoon salt, and sauté for 2 minutes more. Remove from the heat and cover to keep warm.

To serve, divide the spinach between two plates and top each portion with a fish fillet. Serve hot.

Nutrition:

Fat 22g, Carbohydrates 17g, and Protein 19g

21. Quinoa With Curried Black Beans And Sweet Potatoes

Preparation Time: 30 minutes

Cooking Time: 20 minutes

Servings: 2 servings

Ingredients:

½ cup quinoa ½ teaspoon dried rosemary 1 cup of water

1 cup canned black beans, drained ½ cup peeled and diced sweet ½ teaspoon olive oil

One teaspoon mild curry powder potato (about one small) Two tablespoons chopped fresh parsley

Directions:

Rinse the quinoa under cold running water in a fine-mesh sieve. Drain very well over paper towels and then pat dry.

In a small saucepan, toast the quinoa for 2 minutes over medium heat, shaking frequently. Add the water, increase the heat to high, and bring the water to a boil. Cover, reduce the heat to low, and cook for 15 minutes, or until

The quinoa is plump, and the germ forms little spirals on each grain. Remove from the heat and cover to keep warm. In a small bowl, toss the sweet potato with the olive oil and rosemary.

Transfer to a medium skillet over medium-high heat. Sauté, frequently stirring, for 6 to 7 minutes, or until well caramelized. Stir in the black beans and curry powder; reduce the heat to medium, and cook, frequently stirring, until the beans are heated through.

To serve, place ½ cup cooked quinoa on each plate and top with half of the bean mixture. Garnish with the parsley.

Nutrition: Fat 22g, Carbohydrates 17g, and Protein 19g

22. Sirt Fruit Salad

Preparation Time: 10 minutes

Cooking Time: 30 minutes

Servings: 1

Ingredients

½ cup freshly made green tea

1tsp honey

One orange halved

One apple, cored and roughly chopped

Ten red seedless grapes

Ten blueberries

Directions:

Stir the honey into half a cup of green tea. When it's dissolved, add the juice of half the orange. Leave to cool.

Chop the other half of the orange and place in a bowl together with the chopped apple, grapes, and blueberries. Pour over the cooled tea and leave too steep for a few minutes before serving.

Nutrition:

Energy (calories): 121 kcal

Protein: 0.75 g Fat: 0.32 g Carbohydrates: 31.87 g

CHAPTER 4:

Mains

23.   Salad In Four Variations

Preparation time: 10 minutes

Cooking time: 25 minutes

Servings: 4

Ingredients:

50g rocket salad

50g chicory

40g green celery stalk, sliced

20g red onions, sliced

80g avocado, diced

15g walnuts, chopped

1 Medjool date, pitted and chopped

10g parsley, chopped

10g lovage or celery leaves, chopped

One tablespoon of olive oil

One tablespoon capers

1/4 lemon, the juice of which

Directions:

As a base, arrange the chicory and rocket in a bowl. Add all other ingredients and mix well.

The standard addition is 100 g of smoked salmon cut into strips.

For vegans, the salmon can be replaced by 100 g of cooked lentils.

If you prefer meat, use 100 g chopped chicken breast fillet.

If you do not like salmon, you can use 100 g of tuna instead (canned, in your juice).

Nutrition:

Energy (calories): 812 kcal

Protein: 6.61 g

Fat: 72.86 g150%

Carbohydrates: 41.15 g

24.   Waldorf Salad

Preparation time: 10 minutes

Cooking time: 15 minutes

Servings: 4

Ingredients:

100g green celery, roughly chopped

50g apple, roughly chopped

50g walnuts, roughly chopped

10g red onions, roughly chopped

5g parsley, finely chopped

One tablespoon capers

5g lovage (fresh)

One tablespoon of extra virgin olive oil

One teaspoon balsamic vinegar

Juice of a 1/4 lemon

One teaspoon Dijon mustard

50g rocket salad

35g chicory salad

Directions:

Mix celery, apple, walnuts, onions, capers, parsley, and lovage.

Mix a dressing of olive oil, balsamic vinegar, lemon juice, and mustard and briefly marinate the previous ingredients.

Arrange the chicory and rocket on a plate and place the Waldorf salad on top.

Nutrition:

Energy (calories): 805 kcal

Protein: 10.15 g

Fat: 76.67 g

Carbohydrates: 26.58 g

25.   Bean Stew

Preparation time: 10 minutes

Cooking time: 25 minutes

Servings: 1

Ingredients:

One tablespoon of extra virgin olive oil

50g red onions, finely chopped

30g carrots, peeled and finely diced

30g celery stick, finely diced

One clove of garlic, very finely chopped

1/2 Thai chili (red), finely chopped

One teaspoon mixed Italian herbs

One tablespoon of tomato paste

200ml vegetable broth

One tin of small tomatoes (400ml)

200g mixed beans from the tin

50g kale, roughly chopped

One tablespoon parsley, coarsely chopped

40g buckwheat

Directions:

Heat the oil at low heat and add onion, carrot, celery, garlic, chili, and herbs—all sweat.

Add the stock, tomatoes, and tomato paste. Put the beans in and cook for about 30 minutes.

In the meantime, prepare the buckwheat.

Add the kale to the stew, continue cooking for 5 minutes, then sprinkle with parsley and serve.

Nutrition:

Energy (calories): 337 kcal

Fat: 9.08 g

Carbohydrates: 52.54 g

CHAPTER 5:

Meat

26.   Sirtfood Beans With Beef

Preparation Time: 10 min.

Cooking Time: 25 minutes

Servings: 2

Ingredients:

Kidney beans, two small cans

Lean beef, minced, 400 g

Buckwheat, 160 g

One finely chopped red onion

One chopped red bell pepper

Two finely chopped bird's eye chili peppers

Canned tomatoes, 800 g

Ground turmeric1 tbsp.

Tomato sauce 1 tbsp.

Cocoa powder, 1 tbsp.

Ground cumin 1 tbsp.

1 tbsp. Extra virgin olive oil

Red wine, 150 ml

½ tbsp. Chopped coriander

½ tbsp. Chopped parsley

Directions:

Over medium heat, fry the onions, chili peppers, and garlic for three minutes. Throw in the spices and mince for another minute. After that, add the beef and red wine. Bring to a boil and let it bubble until the liquid reduces by half. Add the cocoa powder, tomatoes, tomato sauce, and red bell pepper. Add more water if needed and let the dish simmer on low, medium heat for an hour. Add the remaining chopped herbs before serving.

Nutrition: Energy (calories): 209 kcal Protein: 5.72 g

Fat: 8.16 g

Carbohydrates: 31.8 g

CHAPTER 6:

Sides

27. Baked Potato

Preparation Time: 5 minutes

Cooking Time: 25 minutes

Servings: 4

Ingredients:

4 Russet potatoes (medium-sized, scrubbed)

1 cup of water

Directions:

Pour the water into the inner pot of your Instant Pot. Place the trivet inside the jar.

Using a fork to pierce, poke holes all over the potatoes. Place the potatoes on the trivet in the pot. If the potatoes do not easily fit on the trivet, place an Instant Pot steamer basket on the trivet and then place the potatoes in the basket.

Secure the lid, move the pressure release valve to seal, choose the manual option, and select high pressure. Set the cooking time to 15 minutes.

When the cooking time is completed, allow the pressure to release naturally for 10 minutes. Then, quick release.

Remove the lid.

Use tongs to transfer the potatoes to your dinner plate. Cut the potatoes in half and top with your favorite toppings like cheese, sour cream, or chives.

Nutrition:

Calories 37 Carbs 8.4g Fat 1g Protein 1g

28. Veggie Noodles With Avocado Sauce

Preparation Time: 5 minutes.

Cooking Time: 10 minutes

Servings: 4

Ingredients:

½ pound pumpkin, spiralized

½ pound bell peppers, spiralized

2 tbsp. olive oil

Two avocados, chopped

One lemon, juiced and zested

2 tbsp. sesame oil

2 tbsp. cilantro, chopped

One onion, chopped

One jalapeño pepper, deveined and minced

Salt and black pepper to taste

2 tbsp. pumpkin seeds

Directions:

Toast pumpkin seeds in a dry skillet for a minute, stirring frequently; set aside. Add oil and sauté bell peppers, and pumpkin for 8 minutes. Remove to a serving platter.

Combine avocados, sesame oil, onion, jalapeño pepper, lemon juice, and lemon zest in a food processor and pulse to obtain a creamy mixture. Adjust the seasoning and pour over the vegetable noodles, top with the pumpkin seeds, and serve.

Nutrition: Calories 673 Fat 59 g Carbs 9.8 g Protein 22.9 g

CHAPTER 7:

Seafood

29.   Simple Salmon Dinner

Preparation time: 10 minutes

Cooking time: 25 minutes

Servings: 4

Ingredients:

1 pound salmon filet (skin on)

2 tsp. fresh lemon juice

1/2 teaspoon sea salt

1/2 teaspoon organic garlic powder

1/2 teaspoon lemon pepper

Directions:

Heat a skillet over medium heat.

Drizzle lemon juice then adds the seasonings on top of salmon.

Place the salmon on your grill. The skin side of the salmon must be placed at the surface of the grill. Cook for around 5-10 minutes.

Turn the salmon and cook for another 5-10 minutes. Salmon is cooked when the skin pulls off quickly, and the fish is easy to pull apart with a fork. Try not to overcook.

Once you've removed your salmon from the grill, let it sit for a couple of minutes before serving it.

Serve with a lemon slice; it is extra yummy with more lemon juice squeezed on after you cook it! Enjoy!

Nutrition:

(calories): 1572 kcal

Protein: 275.27 g

Fat: 51.88 g

Carbohydrates: 1.87 g

30.   Fish Pie

Preparation time: 10 minutes

Cooking time: 35 minutes

Servings: 4

Ingredients:

1kg sweet potato (large pieces)

2 tsp. rapeseed oil

Two leeks, chopped lengthwise

400ml skimmed milk

One heaped tbsp. plain flour

300g Pollock, cut into cubes

Pinch white pepper

One fish stock cube

25g fresh parsley chopped

One heaped tsp. smoked paprika   ture and marinate in the refrigerator for 1 hour or overnight.Add flour with salt and pepper to a dish. Dredge the marinated salmon lightly with the flour on both sides. In a medium skillet, heat 1-2 tbsp. Of olive oil over medium-high heat. At a time, cook two fillets for 3-4 minutes per side or until brown

Serve with lime wedges or peach salsa.

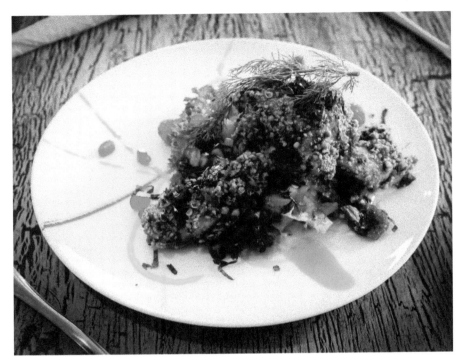

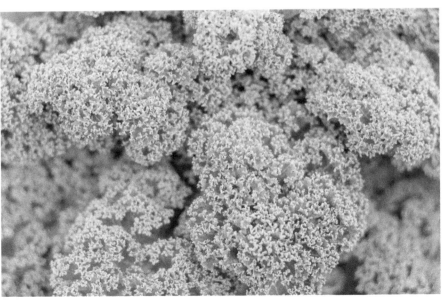

CHAPTER 8:

Poultry

31.   Turkey Meatballs

Preparation time: 10 minutes

Cooking time: 45 minutes

Servings: 4

Ingredients

255g turkey sausage

Two tablespoons of extra virgin olive oil

One can of 425g chickpeas, rinsed and drained

1/2 medium onion, chopped, 2/3 cup

Two cloves of garlic, finely chopped

One teaspoon of cumin

1/2 cup flour

1/2 teaspoon instant yeast for desserts

Salt and ground black pepper

1 cup of Greek yogurt

Two tablespoons of lime juice

Two radicchio hearts, chopped

Hot sauce

Directions:

Preheat the oven to 200°C.

In a food processor, blend the chickpeas, onion, garlic, cumin, one teaspoon salt, and 1/2 teaspoon pepper until all the ingredients are finely chopped. Add the flour, baking powder, and blend to make everything mix well. Transfer to a medium bowl and add the sausage, stirring together with your hands. Cover and refrigerate for 30 minutes.

Once cold, take the mixture in spoonful, forming 1 inch balls with wet hands. Heat the olive oil in a pan over medium heat.

 In two groups, the falafel in the pan and cook until slightly brown, about a minute and a half per side. Transfer to a baking tray and bake in the oven until well cooked, for about 10 minutes.

Mix the yogurt, lime juice, 1/2 teaspoon salt, and 1/4 teaspoon pepper. Divide the lettuce into four plates, season with some yogurt sauce.

CHAPTER 9:

Vegetable

32.   Lettuce Sandwich

Preparation Time: 10 minutes

Cooking time: 15 minutes

Servings: 2

Ingredients:

Four lettuce leaves

3 oz. tofu cheese, cubed

1/3 cup white mushrooms, chopped

2 oz. Cheddar cheese, shredded

Three tablespoons heavy cream

One teaspoon olive oil

One teaspoon salt

One teaspoon ground black pepper

½ teaspoon apple cider vinegar

Directions:

Sprinkle tofu cubes with the apple cider vinegar.

Put the butter and olive oil in the skillet.

Add mushrooms and mix up.

Sprinkle the mushrooms with ground black pepper and mix up.

Cook the vegetables for 5 minutes over medium heat.

Then add cubed tofu and mix up.

Cook the ingredients for 5 minutes more.

Then add heavy cream. Mix up well.

Close the lid and cook the mixture for 3 minutes more.

Fill two leaves with the mushroom mixture, add shredded cheese, and cover with the remaining lettuce leaves.

The sandwiches are cooked.

Nutrition: calories 251 fat 21.9, fiber 1, carbs 3.7, protein 11.6

33.   Cream Broccoli Dip

Preparation Time: 10 minutes

Cooking time: 20 minutes

Servings: 4

Ingredients:

1 cup of coconut milk

1 cup of water one teaspoon salt

¼ cup Cheddar cheese, shredded

½ teaspoon ground black pepper

1 cup broccoli, chopped

½ onion, diced

One teaspoon butter

½ teaspoon chili flakes

Directions:

Pour coconut milk and water into the pan.

Add chopped broccoli and ground black pepper.

Close the lid and start to cook it over medium heat.

Meanwhile, put the butter in the skillet and preheat it.

Add diced onion and cook it for 3 minutes.

Then transfer the onion to the broccoli mixture.

Add chili flakes, salt, and shredded Cheddar cheese.

Stir the mixture with the help of the spoon well.

Then close the lid and simmer it for 5 minutes over low heat.

With the help of the hand blender, blend the mixture.

When it is smooth, pour it into the big bowl and let it chill till room temperature.

Nutrition: calories 189, fat 17.7, fiber 2.3, carbs 6.4, protein 4

34.   Cauliflower Pat

Preparation Time: 15 minutes

Cooking time: 35 minutes

Servings: 6

Ingredients:

1-pound cauliflower head

One tablespoon olive oil three teaspoons butter

¼ cup fresh dill, chopped

One teaspoon salt

Four tablespoons cream cheese

Two pecans, chopped

One teaspoon minced garlic

Directions:

Sprinkle the cauliflower with olive oil and transfer to the oven.

Bake cauliflower for 35 minutes at 360F. Check it during the cooking. The cooked vegetables should be soft.

Meanwhile, put the butter, chopped dill, salt, cream cheese, pecans, and garlic in the food processor.

Process the mixture until it is smooth.

When the cauliflower is cooked, chop it roughly and add it to the food processor.

Blend the mixture for 3 minutes.

Then transfer the cooked pasta to the bowl and flatten its surface with the spoon's help.

Chill it well.

Nutrition: calories 85, fat 6.7, fiber 2.7, carbs 6.1, protein 3

CHAPTER 10:

Soup, Curries and Stews

35. Cold Tomato And Melon Soup

Preparation Time: 10 minutes

Cooking Time: 30 minutes

Servings: 4

Ingredients:

Beef tomato

½ melon

One little bean stew pepper

150 g little ringer pepper (1 little chime pepper)

1 tbsp. juice

500 ml juice

Salt

Pepper

Two spring onions

Four stems mint

4 tsp. vegetable oil

Directions:

Clean and wash diced tomatoes. Divide the melon, evacuate the stones, strip, and cut the mash into shapes, a number of them aside. Divide, cleave, wash, and slash lengthways. Divide the pepper, expel the seeds, clean, and dig 3D shapes.

Put tomatoes, melon, half the solid paprika shapes, and bean stew with lime and tomato squeeze during a blender and puree until a soup-like consistency is acquired, including touch water if necessary. Season everything with salt and pepper and refrigerate for around half-hour.

Within the interim, clean, wash, and cut the spring onions into fine rings. Wash mint, shake dry, pluck leaves, and usually hack.

Divide the soup into four dishes, sprinkle with spring onions, remaining peppers, melons, and mint, shower with one teaspoon of oil

Nutrition:

Energy (calories): 363 kcal

Protein: 7.6 g

Fat: 19.41 g

Carbohydrates: 48.8 g

36. Kale Pork

Preparation Time: 10 minutes

Cooking Time: 30 minutes

Servings: 4

Ingredients

1tbsp. olive oil

1 pound cubed pork tenderloin

3/4 tsp. salt

One medium red onion, finely chopped

Four cloves garlic, minced

Two teaspoons paprika

1/4 tsp. crushed red pepper (optional)

1 cup red wine

Four plum tomatoes, chopped

4 cups chicken broth

One bunch kale, chopped

2 cups cooked white beans

Directions:

Heat olive oil in a pot over (medium/high) heat. Add pork, season with salt, and cook until no longer pink. Transfer to a plate and leave juices in the pot.

Add onion to the pot and cook until it turns translucent.

Add paprika, garlic, and crushed red pepper and cook for about 30 seconds.

Add tomatoes and wine, increase heat and stir to scrape up any browned bits. Add broth. Bring to a boil.

Add kale and stir until it wilts. Lower the heat and simmer until the kale is tender. Stir in beans, pork, and pork juices. Simmer for two more minutes.

37.   Haitian Kale Shrimp Stew

Preparation Time: 10 minutes

Cooking Time: 8 hours

Servings: 8

Ingredients:

2 cups chopped onions

2 tbsp. olive oil

Salt, black pepper to taste

4 pounds shrimp

3 cups kale leaves

1 tsp. Dried red pepper flakes (to taste).

4 whole cloves (discard after cooking)

2 cups fish broth

1 cup tomato paste

1 lime – juice only & 1/8 ground cloves

Direction:

Put ingredients in the slow cooker—cover & cook on low for 8 hours.

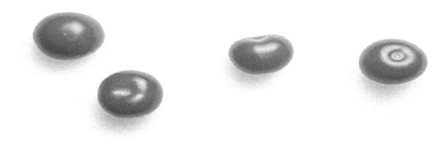

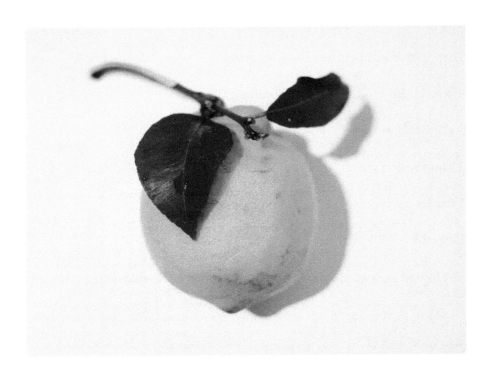

CHAPTER 11:

Snacks & Desserts

38.   Avocado Deviled Eggs

Preparation Time: 10 minutes

Cooking Time: 5 minutes

Servings: 3

Ingredients:

Three eggs

One avocado

One tablespoon chopped chives

One tablespoon freshly squeezed lime juice

Directions:

Peel your hard-boiled eggs and cut them in half, lengthways.

Remove the cooked yolk and add to a mixing bowl along with the avocado and lime juice.

Mash it with a fork until you achieve the desired texture. Stir in the chopped chives.

Either spoon the mixture back into the eggs or pipe it into the eggs using a piping bag or zip lock back.

Serve straight away.

Nutrition: Calories 156 Fat 5.3g Carbohydrates 3.8g Protein 3.4g

39.   Spicy Roasted Nuts

Preparation Time: 20 minutes

Cooking Time: 15 minutes

Servings: 6

Ingredients:

8 oz. pecans or almonds or walnuts

One tablespoon olive oil or coconut oil

One teaspoon paprika powder or chili powder

One teaspoon ground cumin

One teaspoon salt

Directions:

Mix all ingredients in a medium frying pan, and cook on medium heat until the almonds are warmed.

Let cool and serve as a snack with a drink. Store it in a container with a lid at room temperature.

Nutrition: Calories 201 Fat 7g Carbohydrates 5g Protein 4g

40. Crab Salad Stuffed Avocado

Preparation Time: 15 minutes

Cooking Time: 10 minutes

Servings: 2

Ingredients:

4 oz. lump crab meat

Two tablespoons light mayonnaise

One teaspoon chopped fresh chives

¼ cup peeled and diced cucumber

Two teaspoons Sriracha, plus more for drizzling

One small avocado (about 4 oz. avocado when pitted and peeled)

½ teaspoon furikake

Two teaspoons gluten-free soy sauce

Directions:

In a medium bowl, combine mayonnaise, Sriracha, and chives. Add crab meat, cucumber, and chive and gently toss. Cut the avocado open, remove the pit and peel the skin or spoon the avocado out. Fill the avocado halves equally with crab salad. Top with furikake and drizzle with soy sauce.

Nutrition: Calories 194 Fat 13g Carbohydrates 7g Protein 12g

41.   Cheddar Olive

Preparation Time: 15 minutes

Cooking Time: 20 minutes Servings: 6-8

Ingredients:

- 1 8-10 jar pitted olives, either pimento-stuffed or plain

- 1 cup all-purpose flour

- 1 ½ cups shredded sharp cheddar cheese

- ¼ teaspoon freshly grated black pepper

- 4 tablespoons unsalted butter, softened

Directions:

Preheat oven to 400° F. Drain the olives well and dry them thoroughly with clean dish towels. Set aside.

Combine the cheese, flour, butter, and spices in a medium bowl and knead it within the bowl until a dough form. If the dough is still crumbly and won't hold together, add water one teaspoon at a time until it does.

Pinch off a small amount of dough, and press it as thin as you can between your fingers to flatten. Wrap it and kiss the dough around a dry olive. Pinch off any excess, and then roll the olive in your hands until smooth. Continue until all the olives are covered. Bake for 15-20 minutes, or until golden brown all over. Serve immediately and enjoy!

Nutrition: Calories 195 Fat 12.2gCarbohydrates 8.1g Protein 6.9g

42.   Crispy Breaded Tofu Nuggets

Preparation Time: 15 minutes

Cooking Time: 20 minutes

Servings: 4

Ingredients:

One block extra firm tofu

1 cup panko bread crumbs

Two flax eggs let sit 5 minutes before using

½ cup vegetable broth

One tablespoon lite soy sauce

½ cup all-purpose flour

1 ½ teaspoons paprika

½ teaspoon onion powder

½ teaspoon garlic powder

½ teaspoon cayenne pepper

¼ teaspoon salt

¼ teaspoon fresh ground black pepper

Directions:

Preheat oven to 400° F. Line a baking sheet with parchment paper.

Slice the tofu into ten squares. Cut the tofu into five slices along the long edge, and then cut each column in half to make squares. Lightly press each piece of tofu with a paper towel to remove some of the liquid.

To make the marinade, stir together the vegetable broth and soy sauce in a shallow pan. Marinate the tofu in the vegetable broth mixture for at least 10 minutes.

Prepare three bowls: one with the flour, one with panko bread crumbs and spices, and one with the flax eggs. Coat the tofu in the flour, then the flax eggs, and finally the panko

Bake at 400° F on the parchment-lined baking sheet for 15 minutes. Carefully flip the tofu bites over, and then bake for another 15 minutes. They're ready when golden brown and crispy. Enjoy!

Nutrition: Calories 127 Carbohydrates 23g Protein 5g

43.　Rosemary Toasted Walnuts

Preparation Time: 10 minutes

Cooking Time: 20 minutes

Servings: 8

Ingredients:

2 cups raw walnuts

Two tablespoons fresh rosemary, finely chopped

¼ cup olive oil

½ teaspoon salt

One teaspoon pepper

Directions:

Preheat oven to 350° F. Line a baking sheet with parchment paper.

In a bowl, whisk together olive oil, rosemary, salt, and pepper.

Add in walnuts and toss until completely covered in olive oil mixture. Bake the walnuts for 10-15 minutes in the oven, tossing every 4-5 minutes until their golden brown. The walnuts cook quickly, so be careful not to burn them. Enjoy!

Nutrition: Calories 223 Fat 23g Carbohydrates 5g Protein 4g

CHAPTER 12:

Desserts

44.   Peanut Butter Truffles

Preparation Time: 10 minutes

Cooking Time: 30 minutes

Servings: 4

Ingredients:

5 tbsp. peanut butter

1 tbsp. coconut oil

1 tbsp. raw honey

1 tsp. ground vanilla bean

¾ cup almond flour

Coating:

Pinch of salt

1 cocoa butter

½ cup 70% chocolate

Directions:

Mix the peanut butter, c all ingredients into a dough.

Roll out the dough into 1-inch balls, lay them on parchment paper, and refrigerate for half an hour (you get about 12 truffles).

Melted chocolate and cocoa butter, add a pinch of salt. Dip each truffle in the melted chocolate, one at a time. Put them back on the baking sheet with parchment paper and put them in the fridge.

Nutrition: Calories: 194 Fat: 8g Carbohydrate: 13.1g Protein: 4g

45.   Chocolate Pie

Preparation Time: 10 minutes

Cooking Time: 30 minutes

Servings: 4

Ingredients:

2 cups flour

1 cup dates, soaked and drained

1 cup dried apricots, chopped

1½ tsp. ground vanilla bean

Two eggs

One banana, mashed

Five cocoa powder

Three raw honey

One ripe avocado, mashed

2 tbsp. organic coconut oil

½ cup almond milk

Directions:

In a bowl, combine the flour, finely chopped apricots, and dates and mix. Add the banana and lightly beaten eggs and mix.

Add the vanilla, cocoa, honey, avocado, and coconut oil and mix.

Gradually add the almond milk. It may take less than ½ cup to get the right "pie texture."

Place in a greased pan and bake for 30-35 minutes at 350 ° F. Always check the cake and leave a few more minutes if it is not cooked.

Allow cooling before serving.

Nutrition: Calories: 380kcal Fat: 18.4g Carbohydrate: 50.2g Protein: 7.2g

46.   Chocolate Walnut Truffles

Preparation Time: 10 minutes

Cooking Time: 35 minutes

Servings: 4

Ingredients:

1 cup ground walnuts

1 tsp. cinnamon

½ cup of coconut oil

¼ cup raw honey

Two chia seeds

Two cacao powder

Direction:

Mix all the ingredients and prepare the truffles.

 Cover with cinnamon, coconut flakes, or ground almonds.

Nutrition:

Calories: 120kcal

Fat: 4.4g

Carbohydrate: 10.2g

Protein: 5.2g

47.   Frozen Raw Blackberry Cake

Preparation Time: 10 minutes

Cooking Time: 45 minutes

Servings: 4

Ingredients:

Crust:

3/4 cup shredded coconut

15 dried dates soaked and drained

1/3 cup pumpkin seeds

1/4 cup of coconut oil

Coconut whipped cream

Top filling:

1 pound of frozen blackberries

¾ cup raw honey

1/4 cup of coconut cream

Two egg whites

Directions:

Grease the pan with coconut oil and mix all the primary ingredients in the blender until you get a sticky ball. Press the base mixture into a cake pan. Make the coconut whipped cream.

Blend the berries, and then add the honey, coconut cream, and egg whites.

Pour the central filling - Coconut whipped cream and distribute evenly.

Pour the top of the berry mixture into the pan, spread, garnish with blueberries and almonds and return to the freezer.

Nutrition: Calories: 472 Fat: 18g Carbohydrate: 15.8g Protein: 33.3g

48.   Chocolate Hazelnuts Truffles

Preparation Time: 10 minutes

Cooking Time: 30 minutes

Servings: 12

Ingredients:

1 cup ground almonds

1 tsp. ground vanilla bean

½ cup of coconut oil

½ cup mashed pitted dates

12 whole hazelnuts

Two cacao powder

Direction:

Mix all ingredients and make truffles with one whole hazelnut in the middle.

Nutrition: Calories: 70 Fat: 2.8g Net carbs: 16.9g Protein: 2.2g

49.   Chocolate Pudding With Fruit

Preparation Time: 10 minutes

Cooking Time: 45 minutes

Servings: 2

Ingredients:

Chocolate cream:

One avocado

2 tsp. raw honey

2 tbsp. coconut oil

3 tsp. cacao powder

1 tsp. ground vanilla bean

Pinch of sea salt

¼ cup of coconut milk

Fruits:

One chopped banana

1 cup pitted cherries

1 tbsp. coconut flakes

Directions:

Blend all the ingredients of the chocolate cream and divide it into two cups.

Place the fruit pieces on top and sprinkle with grated coconut.

Refrigerate at least 2 hours before serving.

Nutrition: Calories: 106kcal Fat: 5g Carbohydrate: 20.4g Protein: 14g

50.   Chocolate Maple Walnuts

Preparation Time: 15 minutes

Cooking Time: 30 minutes

Servings: 15

Ingredients:

½ cup pure maple syrup,

2 cups raw, whole walnuts

½ cup dark chocolate, at least 85%

1 ½ tbsp. coconut oil, melted

1 tbsp. water

1 tsp. of vanilla extract

Directions:

Line a large baking sheet with parchment paper. In a medium to a large skillet, combine the walnuts and ¼ cup maple syrup and cook over medium heat, continually stirring, until the walnuts are completely coated in syrup and golden in color, about 3 - 5 minutes.

Pour the walnuts onto the parchment paper and separate them into individual pieces with a fork. Allow complete cooling; at least 15 minutes.

Meanwhile, melt the chocolate with the coconut oil, add the remaining maple syrup and mix until blended. When the nuts have cooled, transfer them to a glass bowl and pour the melted chocolate syrup over them.

Mix with a silicone spatula until the walnuts are gently covered.

Transfer back to the baking sheet, lined with parchment paper, and separate each of the nuts with a fork.

Put nuts in the refrigerator for 10 minutes or in the freezer for 3-5 minutes, until the chocolate has completely solidified.

Store in an airtight bag in your refrigerator.

Nutrition: Calories 139 Fat 10 g Carbohydrate 19 g Protein 24 g

51.　Matcha And Chocolate Dipped Strawberries

Preparation Time: 25 minutes

Cooking Time: 25 minutes

Servings: 5

Ingredients:

4 tbsp. cocoa butter

Four squares of dark chocolate,

¼ cup of coconut oil

1 tsp. Matcha green tea powder

20 – 25 large strawberries, stems on

Directions:

Melt the cocoa butter, dark chocolate, coconut oil, and Matcha until smooth. Remove from heat and continue stirring until the chocolate is completely melted.Pour into a large glass bowl and stir continuously until the chocolate thickens and begins to lose its luster, about 2 - 5 minutes.One at a time, hold the strawberries by the stems and dip them into the matcha chocolate mixture to coat them. Let the excess drip back into the bowl.Place on a baking sheet lined with parchment paper and cool the dipped berries in the refrigerator until the shell has solidified, 20-25 minutes.

Nutrition: Calories 188 Fat 5.3 g Carbohydrate 10.9 g Protein 0.2 g

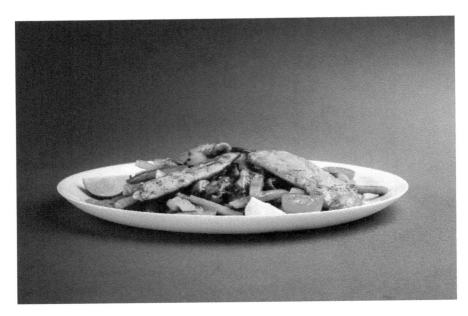

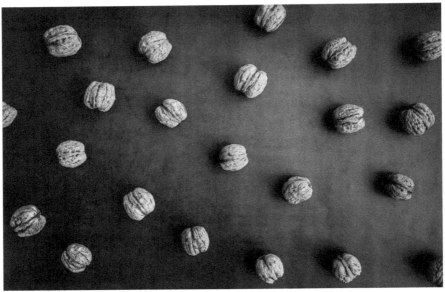

Conclusions

Most diets have been proven to be just a temporary fix. If you want to keep weight off for a good while maintaining muscle mass and ensuring that your body stays healthy, then you need to be following a diet that activates your sirtuin genes: in other words, the Sirtfood Diet.

It is essential to eat a diet that combines whole, healthy, nutritious ingredients with various sirtfoods. These ingredients will all work together to increase the bioavailability of the sirtfoods even further. And there's no need to count calories: just focus on sensible portions and consume a diverse range of foods—including as many sirtfoods as you can and eating until you feel full.

You should also ensure you have a green sirtfood-rich juice every day to get all of those sirtuins- activating ingredients into your body. Also, feel free to indulge in tea, coffee, and the occasional glass of red wine. And most importantly, be adventurous. Now is the time to start leading a happy, healthy, and fat-free life without having to deprive you of delicious and satisfying food.

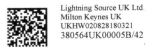

Lightning Source UK Ltd.
Milton Keynes UK
UKHW020828180321
380564UK00005B/42